Baby Chronicles

presents

W9-AAR-401

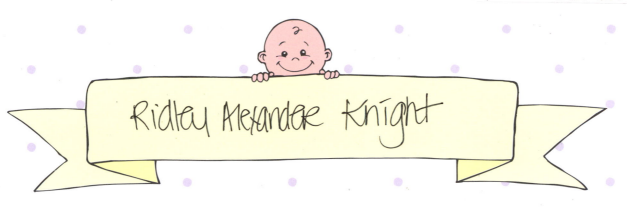

Ridley Alexander Knight

Attach hospital or newborn
baby picture here

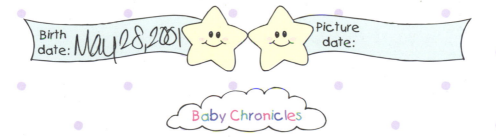

Birth
date: May 28, 2001

Picture
date:

Baby Chronicles

Table Of Contents

 Ready Or Not

Here I Come

First Things First

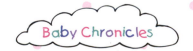
Baby Chronicles

Table Of Contents

I'm A Big Kid Now

Medical History & Development

I'm Number One

Parent's Section

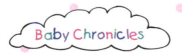

Mommy's Pregnancy Records

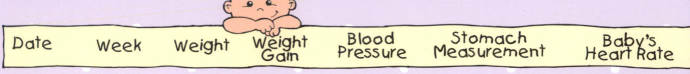

Date	Week	Weight	Weight Gain	Blood Pressure	Stomach Measurement	Baby's Heart Rate
			← Beginning weight			

Record prenatal movements. Include Baby's first heartbeat, first hiccup, first kick…
Take notes on the pregnancy. Include details like Mommy's food cravings, heartburn,
nausea, whether you knew gender of Baby in utero, amniocentesis…

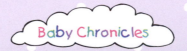
Baby Chronicles

Expecting Company

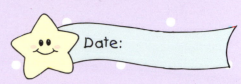
Date:

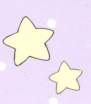

Picture of Mommy Pregnant with Me

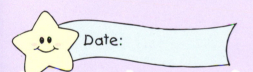
Date:

Picture of Family Before I Arrived

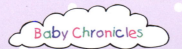

My Ultrasound / Sonogram

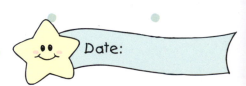

Date:

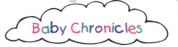

Baby Chronicles

Family & Friends To Notify

Name	Telephone Number	E-mail Address

List of people my parents want
to notify about my birth

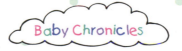

My Arrival

Name Ridley Alexander Knight

Named after great grandfather Alex Parks

Almost named

Date May 28, 2001

Time 6:50 pm

Place Meridian Park Hospital Tualitan, OR

Weight 6 pounds 12 ounces

Height 20½ inches

Head measurement 13 inches

Apgar score 8/9

Eye color Hazel

Hair color Sandy blond

Blood type

Birthmarks

Doctor (delivery) Midwife - Molly Strattan

Doctor (obs/gyn)

Original due date June 4, 2001

Days early/late 1 week early

Natural/ceasarean Natural - no drugs

Drugs during birth

Labor (hours) about 14 hours

Stay in hospital (days) 2 days

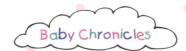

Ask your doctor(s) to autograph here

Hospital I.D.

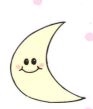

Mine

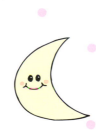

My Parents

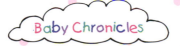

My Birth Announcement

Date _____

Newspaper _____

City _____

Attach newspaper birth
announcement and
birth announcement
cards sent out

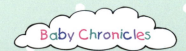
Baby Chronicles

My Birth Certificate

Attach photocopy of birth
certificate or birth card

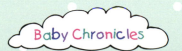

My Horoscope

Birth Sign _____

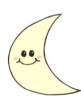

My Birthday Horoscope

Attach horoscope from
newspaper

Date _____

Newspaper _____

City _____

Baby Chronicles

Sign Of The Times

Family car(s) (year, color, model) Mom's - Lexus LX470 - 1998
Dad's - X5 BMW

World Leaders Pres. George W. Bush, V.P. Dick Cheney

Stock market index/currency rate _____
Price of newspaper _____
Price of milk _____
Price of a loaf of bread _____
Price of a chocolate bar _____
Price of gasoline _____
Price of diapers _____
Cost of using a payphone _____

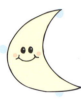

Sample of Postage Stamps

Attach postage stamps

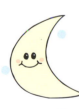

Sample of Dollar Bill or Coin Issued/Used This Year

Attach dollar bills or coins

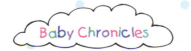

Prime Time News

Newspaper Headlines on the Day I Was Born

Attach newspaper clipping

Date _____

Newspaper _____

City _____

14

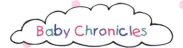
Baby Chronicles

Other News & Forecasts

Date _____

Newspaper _____

City _____

Attach other memorable
pages of the newspaper

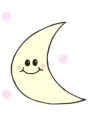

Temperature

Record the weather on day of Baby's birth.
Detail whether windy, snowy, rain or shine

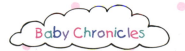

My Family Tree

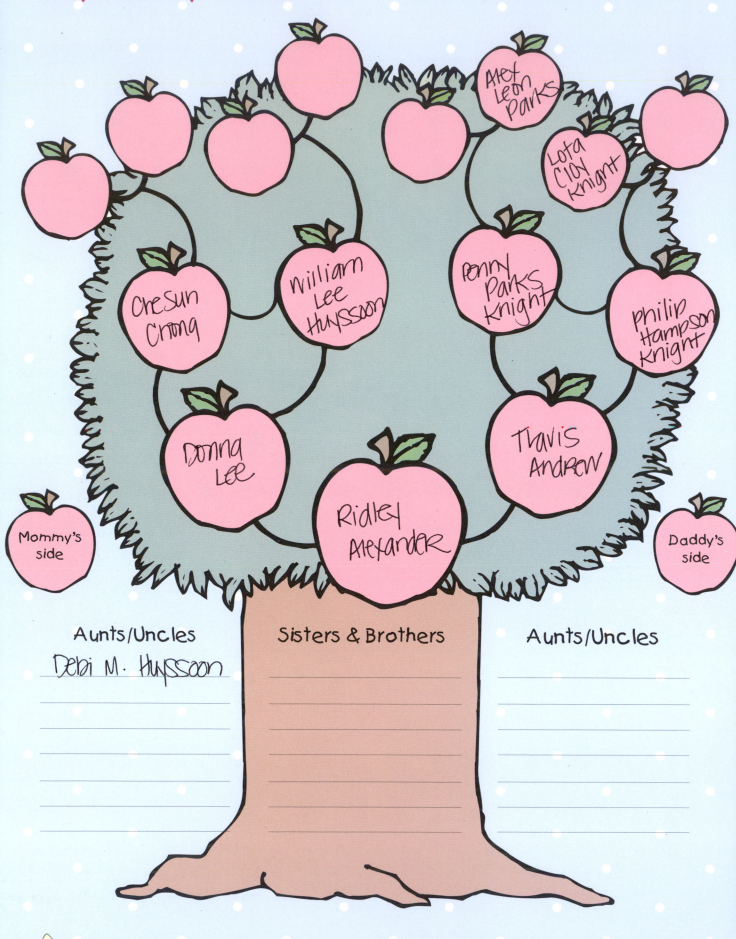

Alex Leon Parks

Lota Cion Knight

Che Sun Chong

William Lee Huyssoon

Penny Parks Knight

Philip Hampson Knight

Donna Lee

Travis Andrew

Ridley Alexander

Mommy's side

Daddy's side

Aunts/Uncles	Sisters & Brothers	Aunts/Uncles
Debi M. Huyssoon		

Baby Chronicles

My Family Close-up

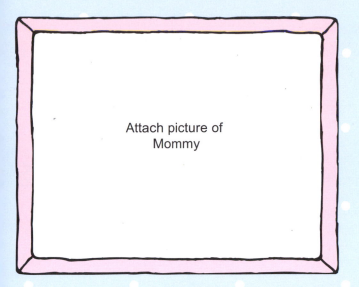

Attach picture of
Mommy

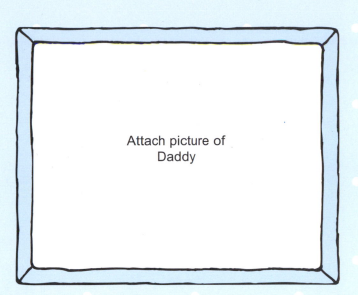

Attach picture of
Daddy

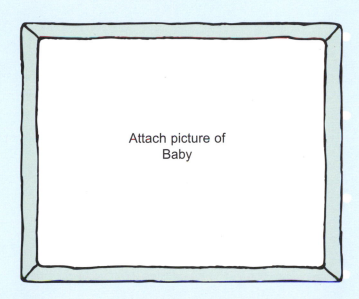

Attach picture of
Baby

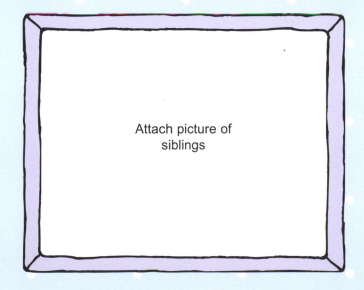

Attach picture of
siblings

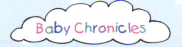

Baby Chronicles

17

My Family Portraits

Photographs with Family and Special Friends

_____

_____

_____

List Baby's cousins, friends...

Home Sweet Home

Address   34645 SW Cloudcrest Lane

Hillsboro, OR 97123

Telephone Number (503) 628· 2170

E-mail Address

My Bedroom

Attach picture of
Baby's bedroom

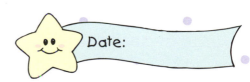

Date:

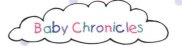

Celebrating My Arrival

Attach picture taken at baby
naming or other ceremony

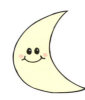 Parent's Notes

 Record name of ceremony, date, time,
place, those officiating, special honors …

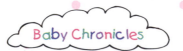

My Autograph Page

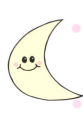

Collect Autographs

Ask visitors to sign their names and
to write a few personal words to Baby

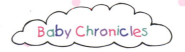

My Presents

From	Gift	Thank You

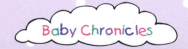

My Presents...

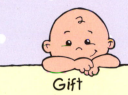

From	Gift	Thank You

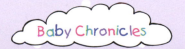

My First

	Date	Age	Comments

No Talk

	Date	Age	Comments
Belly button cord falls off			
First bath in baby tub			
First bath in real tub			
First walk in stroller			

Table Talk

	Date	Age	Comments
Introduced a bottle			
Introduced formula			
First fruit juice			
Holds bottle			
If nursing, weaning began			
If nursing, weaning ended			
Drinks from a cup			
Drinks from a straw			
Drinks milk			
Feeds self (hands)			
Feeds self (spoon)			
Throws food			

Pillow Talk

	Date	Age	Comments
Sleeps in a cradle			
Sleeps in a crib			
First long sleep through night			
Regularly sleeps through night			
Rubs eyes when tired			
Stands in crib			
Climbs out of crib			
Sleeps in a regular bed			

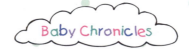
Baby Chronicles

My First...

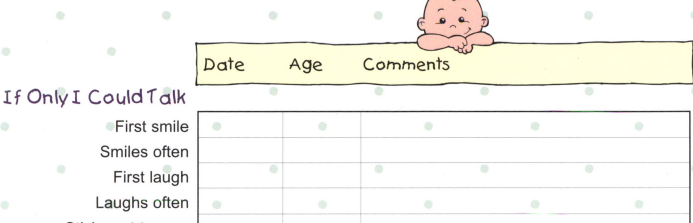

	Date	Age	Comments

If Only I Could Talk

	Date	Age	Comments
First smile			
Smiles often			
First laugh			
Laughs often			
Sticks out tongue			
Makes pleasant sounds			
Shakes head (no)			
Nods head (yes)			
Waves hello/goodbye			
First word			
Talks			

Body Talk

Head

	Date	Age	Comments
Lifts head			
Loses hair			

Hands

	Date	Age	Comments
Sucks thumb			
Plays with feet			
Holds rattle or toy			
Reaches out to parent			
Reaches for things			
Points			
Claps			

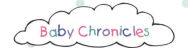

My First...

	Date	Age	Comments

Body

	Date	Age	Comments
Rolls from tummy			
Rolls from back			
Rests on elbows			
Goes on hands & knees			

Tush

	Date	Age	Comments
Sits alone			
Goes into sitting position			
Uses child carseat*			
Uses booster carseat*			
Outgrows carseat*			
Uses highchair			
Uses booster seat at table			
Sits in chair (without booster)			

Legs

	Date	Age	Comments
Crawls or creeps			
Pulls into standing position			
Crawls up stairs			
Crawls down stairs feet first			
Cruises around furniture			
Stands alone			
First steps			
Walks with help			
Walks alone			
Walks up stairs			

* Ensure child is properly restrained at all times

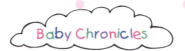
Baby Chronicles

My First...

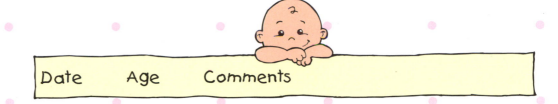

Date	Age	Comments

Potty Talk

Starts potty training		
Makes pee in potty/toilet		
Makes poo in potty/toilet		
Sleeps without diaper		
Fully toilet trained		

More Talk

First day of child care		
First day of pre-school		
First day of kindergarten		
First ride on bus		
Rides tricycle alone		
Rides bicycle		
Talks on telephone		

Record any other memorable firsts

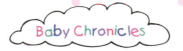

My Hand & Foot Prints

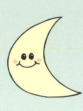

Trace My Hands & Feet at Birth and A Year

Use a pen to trace Baby's hands and feet or get actual prints by using non-toxic, washable paint

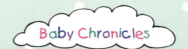

It's Bathtime!

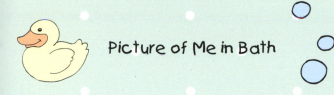

Picture of Me in Bath

Date:

Hint to parents: Think TWICE before inserting truly embarrassing photos!

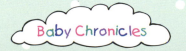

My First Hairdo & Haircut

Date _____

Age _____

Hairdresser _____

Attach Baby's hair

Attach Baby's hair

Save clippings from later haircuts if
Baby's hair color or texture is changing

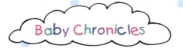

My Before & After Shots

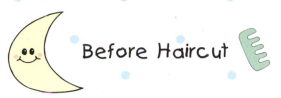

Before Haircut

Date:

Attach picture of Baby
before haircut

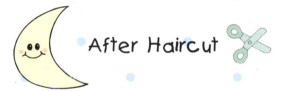

After Haircut

Date:

Attach picture of Baby
after haircut

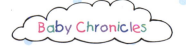

My Introduction To Solid Foods

Solid Foods		Date	Age	Reactions, if any
Cereal (4 mos)	rice			
	barley			
	oatmeal			
Vegetables (5 mos)	peas			
	carrots			
	sweet potatoes			
	squash			
	beans			
	corn			
Fruit (6 mos)	apples			
	bananas			
	peaches			
	pears			
	apricots			
	prunes			
	plums			
Meat (7 mos)	veal			
	chicken			
	turkey			
	beef			
	lamb			
	liver			
Dairy (9 -12 mos)	egg yolk			
	yogurt			
	cottage cheese			
	cheese			
	custard			
Teething Biscuits (9 -12 mos)				

Breast milk or infant formula provides the best form of nutrition for your child during the first year. Usually, infants do not require solids before 4 months of age. When solids are introduced, it is best to introduce them one at a time, several days apart, in the above order. Please consult Baby's pediatrician and follow his/her recommendations on introducing solids.

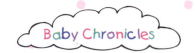

My Food Reviews

Age	Yummy Foods	Yucky Foods

Attach picture of Baby eating

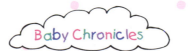

My First Words

Date	Age	Words, Sentences, Funny Phrases, Songs

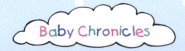
Baby Chronicles

Me And My Friends

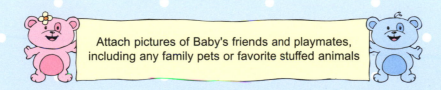

Attach pictures of Baby's friends and playmates, including any family pets or favorite stuffed animals

My First Holiday Season

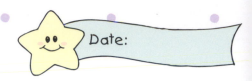
Date:

Attach pictures of Baby celebrating
first festive holiday

Record names of special people
who celebrated with Baby

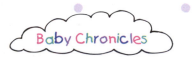
Baby Chronicles

My First Vacation

Date:

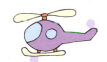

Attach picture of Baby on first vacation.

My Travels

Save travel stubs and souvenirs

Date	Age	Where I Went	How I Got There	Length of Trip

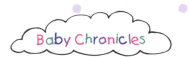

Nicknames & Aliases

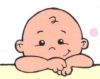

Age	Nickname
Pre-birth	

My Favorite Toys & Books

Age	Toys & Books (Stories)

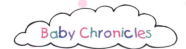

My Scribbles

Date:

Attach some of Baby's first
pieces of artwork

Circle one:

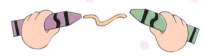

Left handed   Right handed

Date	Signature

Get Baby to sign own name. Do this every
year to see development in writing style

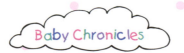

My Portrait Gallery

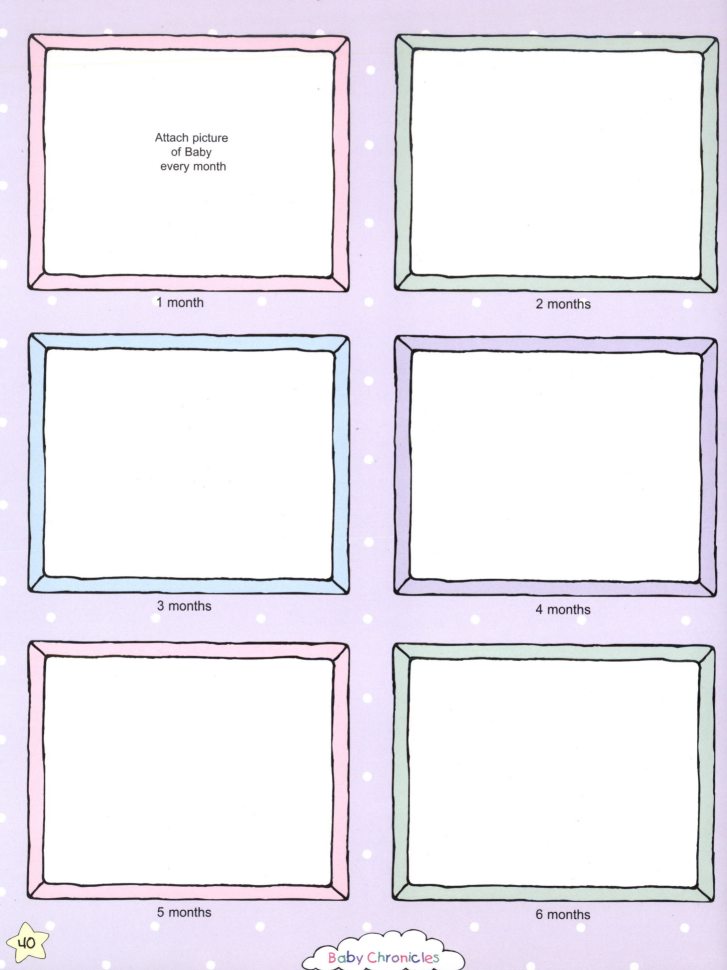

Attach picture
of Baby
every month

1 month

2 months

3 months

4 months

5 months

6 months

Baby Chronicles

My Portrait Gallery...

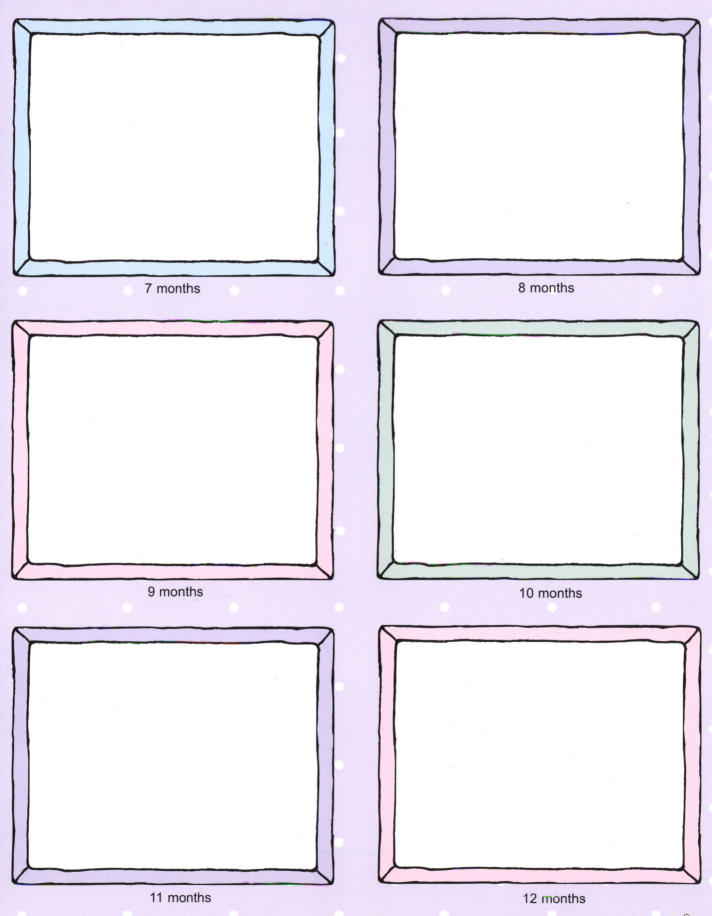

7 months

8 months

9 months

10 months

11 months

12 months

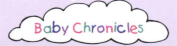

Baby Pictures

 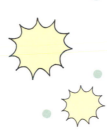 Pictures of Me

 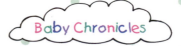 Remember to date all pictures

Baby Pictures...

More Pictures of Me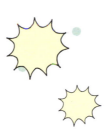

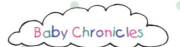

Baby Pictures...

Even More Pictures of Me

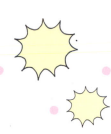

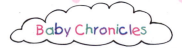

Collectibles

Keep souvenirs like Baby's hospital crib card,
ticket stubs to movies or events...

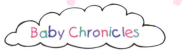

My Growth Chart

Date	Age	Weight	Height

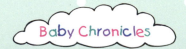
Baby Chronicles

My Growth Graph

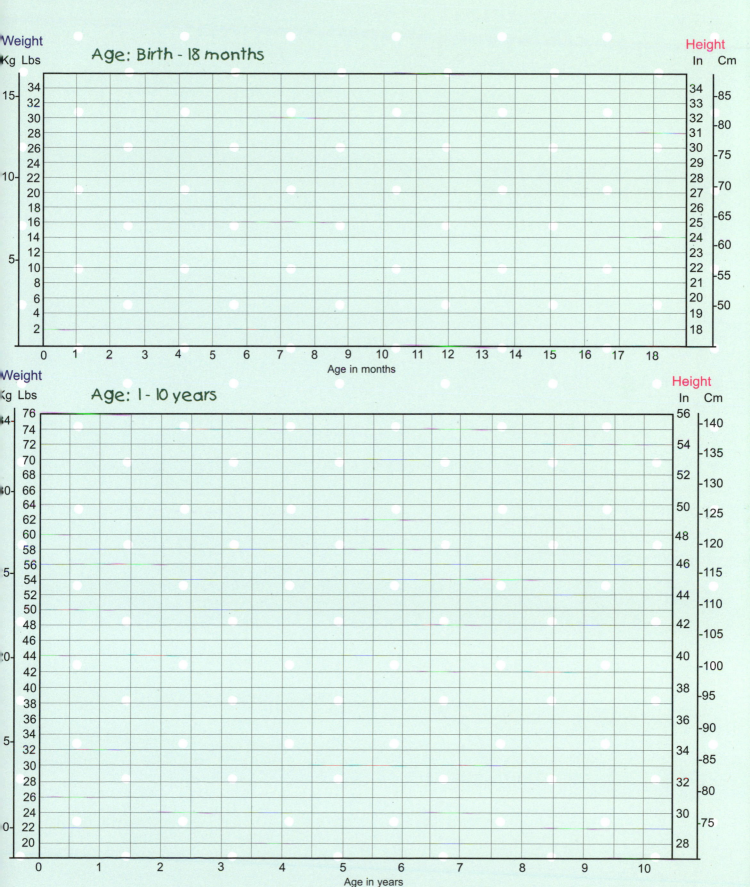

Weight

Age: Birth - 18 months

Height

Age in months

Weight

Age: 1 - 10 years

Height

Age in years

Plot Baby's weight and height measurements from Growth Chart.   Use different color markers each for weight and height.

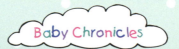

Baby Chronicles

My Medical History

Date	Age	Symptoms, Allergies, Viruses...	Diagnosis & Prescription

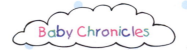
Baby Chronicles

My Immunization Schedule

Date	Age	Vaccine or Booster Injection	Reaction

 ## Recommended Immunization Time Frame

DTP-P	Diphtheria, Tetanus, Pertussis - Polio	2, 4, 6, 18 months, 4 - 6 years
MMR	Measles, Mumps, Rubella	12 - 15 months, 4 - 5 years
TB test	Tuberculin skin test	1 year
Varivax	Chicken pox vaccine	Over 1 year
HIB test	Hemophilus Influenzae Type B	2, 4, 6, 15 - 18 months
Hep. B	Hepatitis B	12 years & over (Canada)
		birth, 1 month, 6 months (U.S.A.)

Please consult your Baby's pediatrician. Photocopy or refer to schedule for school, camp …

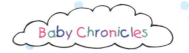 Baby Chronicles

My Baby Teeth

Teething Chart

Record date tooth comes in

1/9/01 ① ← Record order tooth comes in

12/31/06 ② ← Record order tooth falls out

Record date tooth falls out

Top teeth

Picture is Baby's mouth facing you

Bottom teeth

Begin brushing Baby's gums
and teeth at 6 months of age

Baby Chronicles

My Dental Records

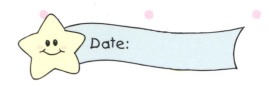

Attach picture of Baby smiling
with new teeth showing

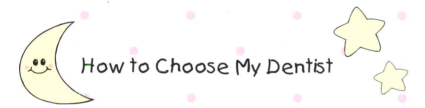 How to Choose My Dentist

Questions

Make a consultation appointment with dentist.
Consider pediatric dentist versus regular dentist.
Does dentist use small instruments for children?
Does dentist have special "incentives" for children?

Comments

Dentist Information

Dentist's name
Dentist's address
Dentist's phone number
Baby's first dentist appointment

Comments

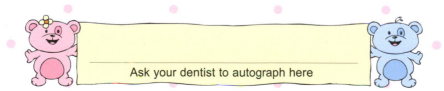
Ask your dentist to autograph here

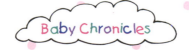

My Tooth Fairy Visits

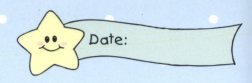

Attach picture of Baby smiling
with some teeth missing

1. Save each tooth in a clear plastic bag
2. Record date tooth falls out on bag
3. Attach bag to this sheet
4. Do the same for each tooth that falls out
5. Save as many teeth as you can

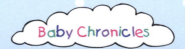
Baby Chronicles

My First Birthday Party

Invitation

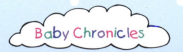

My First Birthday Party...

Date of Party _____
Location _____
Theme _____

Guests	# Adults	# Kids

Total _____

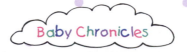

My First Birthday Party...

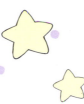

Picture of Birthday Girl/Boy

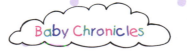

Baby Chronicles

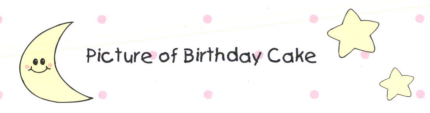

My First Birthday Party...

Picture of Birthday Cake

Attach picture of cake and Baby eating cake

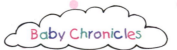

My First Birthday Party...

From	Gift	Thank You

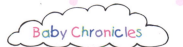
Baby Chronicles

Make Room For Me

Checklist for My Big Arrival

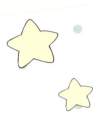

Furniture

- [ ] Bassinet/cradle
- [ ] Crib
- [ ] Baby monitor
- [ ] Diaper-changing table
- [ ] Baby bathtub
- [ ] Dresser drawers
- [ ] Rocking chair
- [ ] Nursery lamp
- [ ] Baby swing
- [ ] Humidifier

Diapers

- [ ] Disposable, cloth diapers or diaper service
- [ ] Baby wipes, lotion, powder
- [ ] Corn starch (to remove carpet stains)
- [ ] Diaper cream & petroleum jelly
- [ ] Diaper pail
- [ ] Facial tissues & cotton balls

Toiletries

- [ ] Thick terry hooded towels
- [ ] Wash cloths
- [ ] Baby shampoo & soap (use baby shampoo as soap)
- [ ] Baby brush & comb
- [ ] Baby nail scissors or clippers
- [ ] Baby thermometer
- [ ] Liquid acetaminophen & saline nose drops

Baby Clothes

- [ ] Undershirts
- [ ] Stretchy terry sleepers
- [ ] Receiving blankets
- [ ] Bunting bag, hat, gloves, socks

Bedding

- [ ] Crib mattress
- [ ] Crib bumper pads
- [ ] Crib sheets
- [ ] Quilted mattress pad (pee pee sheet)
- [ ] Light blankets

Feeding

- [ ] 8 oz bottles
- [ ] 4 oz bottles
- [ ] Extra bottle nipples & caps
- [ ] Breast pump
- [ ] Bottle brushes & liners
- [ ] Bibs
- [ ] Nursing pillow
- [ ] Infant formula

Outings

- [ ] Infant car seat & head hugger
- [ ] Diaper bag
- [ ] Stroller
- [ ] Blanket for stroller

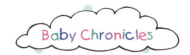
Baby Chronicles

Packing For The Hospital

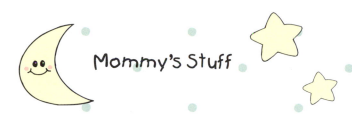

Mommy's Stuff

Labor Bag

- [ ] Medical & hospital cards
- [ ] Bathrobe & slippers
- [ ] Warm socks
- [ ] Pillow & nursing pillow
- [ ] Lollipops, candy ...
- [ ] Snacks for the coach
- [ ] Lip balm or petroleum jelly for dry lips
- [ ] Hand lotion or powder for massage
- [ ] Tennis ball for back pain
- [ ] Facial tissues
- [ ] Eye glasses, contact lenses & solution
- [ ] Magazines, books …
- [ ] Tape recorder & music
- [ ] Camera with film & video camera
- [ ] Small change for telephone
- [ ] Watch or clock
- [ ] Cellular telephone

Overnight Bag

- [ ] Nightgowns that open in front for nursing
- [ ] Underwear
- [ ] Nursing or supportive bras
- [ ] Sanitary pads, breast pads
- [ ] Toiletries (toothbrush, toothpaste, shampoo…)
- [ ] Call list (please see page 7)
- [ ] Nice nightgown for visiting hours
- [ ] Homecoming outfit - loose fitting
- [ ] Baby Chronicles baby book

_____
_____
_____
_____
_____

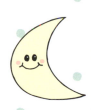

My Stuff

Overnight Bag

- [ ] Baby nail scissors or clippers
- [ ] Diapers, petroleum jelly & facial tissues
- [ ] Baby shampoo & soap (use shampoo as soap)
- [ ] Sleepers, undershirts, socks
- [ ] Receiving blankets

Travel Accessories

- [ ] Bunting bag, hat, sweater, gloves
- [ ] Infant car seat & baby head hugger

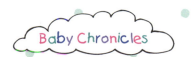

Choosing A Pediatrician

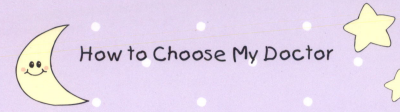

How to Choose My Doctor

Questions

Make a consultation appointment with doctor.
Who recommended doctor?
With what hospitals is doctor affiliated?
Will doctor come to hospital to examine Baby?
Is doctor's office located close to home?
Is there parking available at doctor's office?
What are doctor's office hours?
What is the average waiting time?
Can doctor fit you in if Baby becomes ill?
Is there a group of doctors on call?
How are telephone questions handled?
How are emergencies handled?
Does doctor make house calls?

Comments

Doctor's Information

Doctor's name
Doctor's address
Doctor's telephone number
Consultation date
Back-up doctor

Comments

Ask your doctor to autograph here

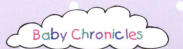

Daily Schedule

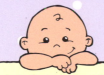

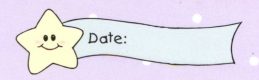

Date:

Time	Feedings	Wet / dirty diapers	Baths	Comments
06:00am				
07:00am				
08:00am				
09:00am				
10:00am				
11:00am				
noon				
01:00pm				
02:00pm				
03:00pm				
04:00pm				
05:00pm				
06:00pm				
07:00pm				
08:00pm				
09:00pm				
10:00pm				
11:00pm				
midnight				
01:00am				
02:00am				
03:00am				
04:00am				
05:00am				

Photocopy this blank schedule and fill in daily until a routine is established.
This schedule is useful:
- to establish a daily pattern for Baby
- to discuss with doctor should any concerns arise
- to leave with babysitter

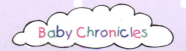

Babysitting Instructions

Our Address

Address _____

Phone # _____ Fax # _____ E-mail _____

Main intersection _____

Directions to our house _____

_____

Parents' full names _____

Kids' names and ages _____

Emergency Phone #'s   911

Doctor _____

Fire _____

Hospital _____

Police _____

Poison Control _____

	Name	Phone #

Work Phone # _____

Friend You Can Call _____

Neighbor _____

- -

Tonight's Destination (place & phone #) _____

Special Instructions _____

_____

_____

_____

_____

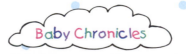

Complete upper portion of this sheet, then make a few photocopies. When parents go out, fill out bottom of one copy and leave with babysitter

Baby Chronicles

Sleeping Patterns

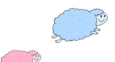

Date	Description

Record Baby's sleeping patterns, naps . . .

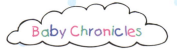

Parent's Notes

Date	Description

Record notes on anything
parents want to remember

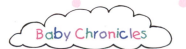
Baby Chronicles

Parent's Notes...

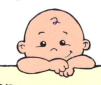

Date	Description

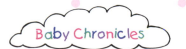

Letters To Baby

Attach letters written by parents, or
other special people, to Baby

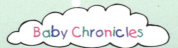
Baby Chronicles

Letters To Baby...

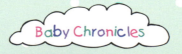

Extras

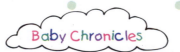